Co

All rights reserved. No reproduced in any form without permission in writing from the publisher except in the case of brief quotations embodied in critical articles or reviews.

Legal & Disclaimer

The information contained in this book and its contents is not designed to replace or take the place of any form of medical or professional advice; and is not meant to replace the need for independent medical, financial, legal or other professional advice or services, as may be required. The content and information in this book have been provided for educational and entertainment purposes only.

You agree that by continuing to read this book, where appropriate and/or necessary, you shall consult a professional (including but not limited to your doctor, attorney, or financial advisor or such other advisor as needed) before using any of the suggested remedies, techniques, or information in this book.

TABLE OF CONTENTS

INTRODUCTION 4

PART ONE: Understanding Crohn Disease 6

    What is Crohn's disease? 6

    Causes of Crohn's Disease 7

    Symptoms of Crohn's Disease 10

PART TWO: LIVING WITH IBD 14

    Dietary Strategies for Managing IBD 14

    The Right Diet 16

    Preventing Malnutrition 19

    Malnutrition Symptoms 20

    Risk Factors 23

    Diet Modifications 24

    Elimination Diets 25

    Exclusion Diet Value 26

    Lactose-Restricted Diets 27

PART THREE: RECIPES 30

Breakfast Recipes..30

Lunch..50

Main Dishes..68

INTRODUCTION

It is extremely important to consider that our relationship with food will affect how we heal. Food is central to the entire chasm of living beings. Practically, food provides nutrients for our body's fuel. It is more central than you may realize. Food stimulates conversations and initiates friendships and relationships. Food is everywhere. Think of how often you may have scheduled a social activity that involved food in one way or another. Dates, having people over, parties, ceremonies, going out after work, going to a friend's house for dinner, lunch meetings, breakfast meetings—these are just a few examples of the many ways that we interact with each other around food.

So why is it that societal food choices are not typically healthy and nourishing? We have veered far from our roots in our food choices and farming practices. Research has shown that poor food choices affect health outcomes for the future. There is a direct correlation between fats, sugars, and processed foods and illness. There is also a direct relationship between healthy foods such as vegetables, fruits, nuts, seeds, and other high-fiber foods and a decrease in negative health outcomes. It is being proven in the research, now we just need to start listening and making changes in our own lives.

As hard as change is, it can be liberating and exhilarating. Increasing healthy foods in your diet is a good start, In this book, you'll discover the realities and challenges of the condition, but also the best treatments, helpful lifestyle changes to help you manage the condition as well as easy and delicious recipes to help relieve your symptoms.

PART ONE: UNDERSTANDING CROHN DISEASE

What is Crohn's disease?

Crohn's disease is a type of inflammatory bowel disease. As many as 780,000 Americans have the condition, according to the Crohn's & Colitis Foundation (CCF).

More research about Crohn's disease is necessary. Researchers aren't sure how it begins, who is most likely to develop it, or how to best manage it. Despite major treatment advances in the last three decades, no cure is available yet.

Crohn's disease most commonly occurs in the small intestine and the colon. It can affect any part of your gastrointestinal (GI) tract, from your mouth to your anus. It can involve some parts of the GI tract and skip other parts.

The range of severity for Crohn's is mild to debilitating. Symptoms vary and can change over time. In severe cases, the disease can lead to life-threatening flares and complications.

Causes of Crohn's Disease

Experts point to a likely combination of genetics, environmental triggers, and a possible imbalance in the microbiome, or gut flora, known as dysbiosis.

• Where You Live: Google Maps could likely spot clusters of Crohn's. Okay, that's a stretch, but seriously: The condition is more common in developed countries than undeveloped countries, in urban cities and towns rather than rural areas, and in northern rather than southern climates. Experts think the latter may be due to lower Vitamin D exposure where it's not as sunny. The usual explanation for the other geographic differences is that people living in less developed areas are exposed to more germs and develop a stronger immune system, but experts are quick to acknowledge that this "hygiene hypothesis" is simplistic at best.

What can't be dismissed is the fact that we are now seeing an increase in Crohn's and ulcerative colitis in places where they were once rare, such as Africa and South Asia, which brings us to the next round of potential triggers. Western habits such as smoking tobacco, eating processed food, and exposure to antibiotics, which are all less common in underdeveloped countries. As areas like these become more modernized, researchers see rates of IBD go up. While we don't yet have research to prove it, it's also worth noting that, anecdotally, clusters of Crohn's have been observed in areas that have been linked to chemical contamination.

- Your Microbiome: Your body is an Airbnb to trillions of microorganisms, including good and bad bacteria. These little guests are known collectively as the microbiome. Many are housed in the gut and digestive tract, along with 70 percent of our immune system. In healthy people, all this gut flora can live together happily. When the balance gets thrown off—which can be due to illness, prolonged use of antibiotics, smoking, or an unhealthy diet—it's known as dysbiosis, a state that has been linked to intestinal disorders.

- Genetics: IBD runs in families, but many people with a family history will never develop it. Studies show that from 5 to 20 percent of IBD patients have a first-degree relative—parent, sibling, or child—with it. The genetic risk is higher for Crohn's than ulcerative colitis, and also significantly higher for either type when both parents have IBD. While Crohn's occurs in people of every ethnic background, it is most common among Caucasians, particularly Jews of eastern European descent. Still, experts believe there is likely more than one gene at work in the development of Crohn's and the majority of people who are diagnosed have no clear family history of IBD.

Symptoms of Crohn's Disease

Most Crohn's patients experience unintended weight loss, and an urgent need to move their bowels, along with the sensation that they're never quite "done" and will need to go again.

And yet, some Crohn's patients defy expectations: They may be over- rather than underweight, and experience constipation, which may be due to medications like iron supplements, pain relievers, and anti-diarrheals; eating too little fiber or too little food in general; not drinking enough water; or an underlying complication such as a stricture or blockage.

Your Crohn's symptoms will depend on where you are in the 3-2-1 cycle. Are your symptoms mild, moderate, or severe? Are you in a flare or are you in remission? In a flare, the disease is at its most active and symptoms are at their worst.

During remission, the disease isn't cured. But the symptoms diminish or go away entirely for a certain amount of time—weeks, months, or years. And the absolute most crucial thing—the first thing, really—you need to determine is the type of Crohn's you may have. So let's start with that number one—the type of Crohn's:

- Ileocolitis: The most common type of Crohn's, Ileocolitis affects the end of the small intestine (known as the terminal ileum) and the colon. Symptoms include diarrhea and cramping, pain in the middle or lower right abdomen, and unintended weight loss.
- Ileitis: This form affects only the small intestine and is also very common. The symptoms are similar to ileocolitis and may include cramping and abdominal pain after meals, diarrhea and unintended weight loss. Patients may also develop fistulas or abscesses in the lower right section of the abdomen.

- Gastroduodenal Crohn's Disease: The stomach and the beginning of the small intestine, known as the duodenum, are affected in this much less common type. Symptoms include nausea, vomiting, loss of appetite, and unintended weight loss.
- Jejunoileitis: This form affects the upper half of the small intestine, known as the jejunum, and is characterized by patchy areas of inflammation in the intestine. Symptoms include abdominal pain and cramps following meals as well as diarrhea. Fistulas may form in more severe cases.
- Crohn's Colitis: This type affects only the colon and causes diarrhea, rectal bleeding, and abscess, fistulas, and ulcers around the anus. Skin lesions and joint pain are also more common with this form. About 20 percent of patients have this type.

Because Crohn's can jump around, affecting the GI tract in patches, some people develop inflammation higher up in the esophagus or mouth. While much less common, when these areas are affected, you might get mouth sores or heartburn, or have chest pain and difficulty swallowing.

Crohn's can sometimes be an out-of-colon experience. The disease can present as extraintestinal (outside the intestines) or systemic symptoms. These occur in up to 36 percent of patients and, like intestinal symptoms, they can be worse during a flare. Some of the more common systemic problems are swollen, painful joints and lower back pain; skin complications like rashes, bumps, and open sores; redness or pain in the eyes and vision changes; fatigue; night sweats; fever; loss of normal menstrual cycle; osteoporosis; and kidney stones.

PART TWO: LIVING WITH IBD

Dietary Strategies for Managing IBD

Nutrition is a topic of high priority not only for people living with Crohn's disease
, but also for their family and friends. Perhaps you have been diagnosed with IBD and are wondering if your current diet is appropriate. Maybe your spouse or child has been diagnosed and you are questioning if the usual foods you buy at the grocery store can still be part of your family's diet. Or maybe you've been living with IBD for a long time but are still afraid to try new foods. How can you find the answers to your questions and, at the same time, feel confident that the information you find is reliable?

Nutrition plays an important role in the management of IBD by maintaining general health during times of disease activity and during times of remission. Diet can also help with symptom management during disease flares. A person's nutritional status affects important physiological processes, such as immunity and wound healing, and, as a result, can contribute to the prevention of long-term complications. Our diet also contributes to our quality of life. Eating good-tasting food that is healthy for you should be your dietary goal, even if you have IBD symptoms. While good nutrition does not cure IBD and while, with certain exceptions, nutritional therapy does not always control disease flares, nutrition is important for health maintenance and symptom management.

Diet Studies

Diet has been studied as a possible cause of Crohn's disease and ulcerative colitis and as a possible treatment for these conditions. Although no one dietary factor has been identified as a cause of IBD, certain dietary factors could possibly play a role in increasing the risk of developing the disease or triggering a disease flare in someone who already has the disease. These factors have not been identified, and no one diet has been proven to cure IBD. Specific foods have been identified as items to avoid in managing some symptoms.

The Right Diet

Many people hear that a particular diet will help their IBD. Gaining a sense of control by changing what or how you eat can be appealing when living with an unpredictable disease. In some cases, the diet may claim to prevent disease relapse or even cure your IBD. Other diets claim to influence your immune system positively, improve digestive health, and reduce inflammation. However, just because it is in print does not mean it is true or scientifically valid.

Sometimes diets are developed in a way that has not been proven or does not even make sense physiologically. It can be difficult to sort out myth from science. A persuasive author or an impressive anecdotal story of someone whose IBD responded only to the author's diet can be very impressive and may leave you with the impression that there is some merit in what the author is suggesting. However, such anecdotes may provide false hope. The money you spend should be for reliable, evidence-based strategies. If you've had difficulty figuring out the "right" diet to follow, it is probably because your experience with diet has been different from someone else's experience.

No IBD Diet

While there is no such thing as an "IBD diet," there are many foods that affect individuals living with IBD adversely or positively. There isn't any single diet that works for everyone with IBD.

Individualized Diets

Accordingly, all nutrition care should be individualized and developed with your doctor or registered dietitian to ensure it is realistic and successful. Remember that Crohn's disease and ulcerative colitis have different parts of the bowel that are inflamed, different disease characteristics, different disease courses, a variety of possible symptoms and possible complications, and variations in treatment regimens.

Nutrition recommendations must be balanced to avoid nutrient deficiencies and individualized to specific tastes, budgets, lifestyles, and, very importantly, for specific desired functional benefits (for example, regaining weight, symptom management). The diet that considers and meets these needs is the right diet for you.

However, there are some common dietary guidelines that people with IBD could follow in an effort to manage their symptoms and improve their quality of life — and even ward off more serious complications, such as malnutrition.

Preventing Malnutrition

Diet is the key for preventing clinical malnutrition, a condition that results when there is a deficiency or imbalance of nutrients in our body. Nutrient deficiencies can result over time from a lack of overall calories (the term "calories" can be used interchangeably with "energy") or from a lack of specific nutrients, such as protein, essential fats, vitamins, minerals, or trace elements.

Malnutrition is a concern because it can affect your immune system function, leading to an increased susceptibility to infections. It also compromises your body's normal defenses against free radicals (damaging molecules produced from pollution, radiation, stress, and smoking), slows down wound healing, and can contribute to long-term complications, such as poor dental health and early bone loss leading to osteoporosis. When you are poorly nourished, the symptoms of your IBD are likely to become more severe or have a more significant impact upon you.

Malnutrition Symptoms

Malnutrition can manifest as weight loss, loss of appetite, muscle weakness (from losing muscle mass), or changes in your skin, hair, nails, gums, eyesight, or mood.

Weight Loss

The most common indicator of malnutrition is a significant loss of body weight. Often, when you are not feeling well, you have little appetite and feel as if you must force yourself to eat. And often you still lose weight despite your efforts. Why does this happen? This is not simply a matter of willpower.

In Crohn's disease and ulcerative colitis, various parts of the gastrointestinal tract become inflamed, and although the inflammation occurs primarily at a local level (the bowel tissue), it can also occur at a whole-body, or systemic, level. Systemic inflammation results from inflammatory molecules (proteins called cytokines), which are produced in the inflamed intestine, but which circulate throughout the body. It is the effect of one or more of these cytokines that can lead to a loss of appetite.

Anorexia is one malnutrition risk factor that, along with other symptoms, such as gastrointestinal intolerance, altered taste, and dietary eliminations (food phobias and dependencies), can lead to inadequate intake. Other risk factors for malnutrition include increased nutrient requirements, malabsorption of nutrients, and increased losses of electrolytes, minerals, trace elements, and proteins. These factors can lead to malnutrition in individuals with IBD, but this doesn't mean that you will develop these symptoms or complications just because you have IBD. Also keep in mind that some are specific to either Crohn's disease or ulcerative colitis.

Anorexia

Loss of appetite and the inability to eat enough to maintain your weight is described as a symptom called anorexia (this term does not mean the same as an eating disorder). Anorexia may be one of the symptoms you experience when your disease is active.

Treatment for Malnutrition

To determine if you are malnourished, health-care professionals will evaluate your symptoms and signs, medical history, height and weight trends, diet history, social and economic circumstances, medications, and laboratory tests. Although there are several complicated formulas that have been developed to evaluate nutritional status and nutritional risk, most physicians and dietitians can answer these questions quite easily. An appropriate nutrition plan can then be created to help manage your illness and achieve your desired health outcomes.

Your nutrition plan could include counseling for diet modifications or implementing specialized nutrition therapies. These could include help with food ideas and also supplementation with nutritional products, replacement of vitamins and minerals, provision of enteral nutrition (liquid nutrition formula delivered using a feeding tube into the stomach or small intestine), or provision of parenteral nutrition (intravenous nutrition infused through a special intravenous line).

Risk Factors

If you experience symptoms or changes similar to those listed among malnutrition risk factors, be sure to mention them to your doctor. The sooner your symptoms are addressed, the less likely you are to experience the negative effects of malnutrition.

Diet Modifications

If your IBD is under control and you live relatively symptom free, there is no need to restrict foods or follow a special diet. Just follow the United States Department of Agriculture (USDA) MyPlate Food Guidance System or Canada's Food Guide. The Dietitians of Canada have also created a Vegetarian Food Guide Rainbow. These reliable diet guides emphasize eating a wide variety of foods that provide the multitude of nutrients your body needs. The key is to select a variety of foods from all food groups in the recommended amounts, with appropriate modifications for vegetarian and vegan diets.

However, if you are experiencing acute disease activity, you may find it helpful to modify your regular diet to help minimize gastrointestinal symptoms, such as cramping, bloating, gas, and diarrhea. Remember that diet plays an important role in maintaining nutritional status, but also in helping with symptom management. It is of utmost importance that dietary changes do not compromise nutritional status or well-being. This means maintaining weight and energy-intake levels, continuing to enjoy eating, and participating in social situations involving food.

Elimination Diets

Elimination diets are popular in the diet industry, and complementary and alternative medicine practitioners may also take this approach to treatment. This type of diet significantly restricts or excludes one or more foods or major food groups. Common examples of exclusions include dairy, wheat or gluten, red meat, yeast, and refined sugars. If you choose to follow an elimination diet, be sure to consider the potential side effects.

Exclusion Diet Value

The value of exclusion diets has not been scientifically proven in IBD. In studies where suspected foods were excluded, individuals didn't experience disease relapse upon reintroduction of the excluded foods.

Side Effects

Consequences of following exclusionary diets over the long term — that is, for more than a few weeks — include possible development of nutrient deficiencies, weight loss, malnutrition, food phobias or obsessions, and a loss of enjoyment of eating. If major food groups are avoided, be sure to speak with a dietitian to learn about alternative foods or supplements for the excluded nutrients.

There is also a psychological danger with elimination diets. Following a diet that claims to control your IBD can contribute to a feeling of being somehow responsible or guilty if your disease becomes active again. Some people feel they may have cheated on the diet because they had difficulty following it exactly, and they are now responsible for their disease coming back. There is no evidence to support this. This type of internalization of responsibility is destructive and takes strength away during a time when it is difficult enough to live with IBD.

If you still feel it is important to try this approach, be sure to set a timeline for evaluating and stopping the dietary eliminations.

Lactose-Restricted Diets

Is there ever a time when it may be appropriate to reduce consumption or avoid a particular food group? When it comes to dairy products, the answer is yes. "Delicious but caution warranted" is a slogan to apply to dairy products if you have IBD. While dairy products are tasty and provide important nutrients, such as protein and calcium, there are specific situations where it may be difficult to digest the primary sugar in milk.

Unless you have a true milk allergy (immune reaction to the protein in milk), there is no danger from eating dairy products. This type of allergy is relatively uncommon. Dairy products do not cause IBD and generally do not result in flares, but you may experience uncomfortable symptoms if you have lactose intolerance and you drink milk or eat dairy products.

Lactose Intolerance

Lactose intolerance is when your body cannot adequately digest the milk sugar lactose.

Lactase Deficiency

Lactose is the principal carbohydrate in dairy products. It is a disaccharide, meaning that it is a larger molecule made up of two smaller sugar molecules, which are the monosaccharides glucose and galactose. An enzyme called lactase in our small intestine is responsible for breaking lactose into glucose and galactose, which are then easily absorbed.

If there is not enough lactase enzyme available to break down lactose into its two smaller sugars, the result is undigested lactose traveling through the small intestine to the large intestine (colon). This is why lactose intolerance can also be correctly called lactase deficiency.

Lactose Intolerance Symptoms

The classic symptoms of lactose intolerance result from undigested lactose traveling through the small bowel and drawing water by osmosis into the bowel, which causes bloating. When the undigested lactose reaches the colon, bacteria ferment it, producing further bloating, cramping, gas, and diarrhea. Symptoms vary among individuals, but typically appear within 30 minutes to several hours after ingestion.

PART THREE: RECIPES

Breakfast Recipes

Slow Cooker Baked Apples

Prep Time: 15 Minutes

Cook Time: 6 Hours

Total Time: 6 Hours 15 Minutes

Servings: 6

Ingredients

- 6 granny smith apples
- 1/4 cup raisins
- 2 tablespoons honey
- Coconut milk to topp

Instructions

1. Core apples. To core, using an apple corer or paring knife, cut around the core (about ¼ inch from the stem all the way around) but leave about half an inch at the bottom. Use the knife to 'drill out' the core.

2. Divide raisins, honey, cinnamon, and coconut oil between the apples.

3. Place apples in a crock pot and add ½ inch of water. Cook on low overnight and enjoy a hot breakfast in the morning!

4. Alternatively, bake covered at 350 degrees in a glass dish for 45 minutes-1 hour in the morning.

5. Top with with cream, yogurt, coconut milk, or just eat plain.

Delicious Overnight Sea Salt and Caramel Coconut Chia Pudding

Prep Time: 10 Minutes

Total Time: 10 Minutes

Servings: 6

Ingredients

- 10 dates pits removed
- 1/2-3/4 cup hot water
- 1 can full fat coconut milk
- 3 tablespoons whole black chia seeds
- 1/2 teaspoon vanilla
- 1/4 teaspoon sea salt

Instructions

1. Cover dates with hot water in your blender container. Allow to sit for a minute to absorb the water (start with 1/2 cup and add another 1/4 cup at the end if too thick).

2. Puree dates and water until a smooth paste forms.

3. Add in coconut milk, chia seeds, vanilla, and sea salt and puree.

4. Pour into one large bowl or 6 small custard cups. Cover, and chill overnight. Enjoy!

Will keep one week in the refrigerator, covered.

Protein-Packed Peanutbutter Banana Mini Muffins

Prep Time: 10 Minutes

Cook Time: 18 Minutes

Total Time: 28 Minutes

Servings: 12 Servings (3 Muffins Each)

Calories: 187 Kcal

Ingredients
- 4 Very ripe with spots Bananas, mashed

- 4 eggs
- 1/4 cup honey
- 1 teaspoon vanilla
- 3/4 cup peanutbutter or almondbutter
- 1/3 cup coconut flour
- 1/4 teaspoon cinnamon
- 1/2 teaspoon baking soda
- 1/4 teaspoon sea salt
- 1/2 teaspoon apple cider vinegar

Instructions

1. Preheat oven to 350 degrees. Place mini muffin liners in a mini muffin pan. Mix the bananas and eggs with a fork in a bowl or in a stand mixer or in a food processor until mixed well. Add honey, vanilla, penautbutter, coconut flour, and cinnamon. Mix well until consistent throughout. Add baking soda, sea salt, and apple cider vinegar and mix one more time.

2. Add to prepared muffin pan, filling 3/4 full (or a touch more). Bake for 18 minutes for the mini muffins, 25 for regular-sized muffins. They are done when they

spring back when pushed on, cook for an additional 2-3 minutes if they dent when pushed after baking.

Coconut Flour Blueberry Banana Breakfast Bars

Prep Time: 10 Minutes

Cook Time: 30 Minutes

Total Time: 40 Minutes

Servings: 16

Ingredients
- 4 bananas very ripe with spots
- 7 eggs preferably pastured
- 4 tablespoons coconut oil
- 2 tablespoons honey
- 2 teaspoons vanilla
- 1 cup coconut flour
- 1 teaspoon baking soda
- 1/2 teaspoon sea salt
- 6 – 8 ounces of fresh or frozen blueberries organic if possible

Instructions

1. Puree the bananas in a food processor or blender, then add the eggs and continue to process until well mixed. Add honey, oil, and vanilla. Blend well. Add flour, baking soda and salt and blend until smooth. Pour batter into a mixing bowl and add the blueberries, stirring well.

2. Grease a 9x13 pan and line it with parchment paper. Pour batter into the pan and bake at 325 degrees Fahrenheit for 30 minutes. Check the bars to see if the top is getting too brown at this point. If it is, cover it with tin foil then continue to bake the bars for 10 more minutes.

Homemade Coconut-Apricot Protein Bar

Prep Time: 15 Minutes
Cook Time: 12 Hours
Total Time: 12 Hours 15 Minutes
Servings: 10

Ingredients
- 1.5 cups about 12 large dates, pits removed)

- 1/2 teaspoon sea salt
- 1/2 cup crispy almonds see how to make here
- 1/2 cup crispy cashews purchase cashew pieces to save money
- 5 scoops 10 tablespoons Collagen Powder (NOT GELATIN)
- 1 cup dried apricots find additive-free dried apricots here. Note: If there aren't additives, oxidation will cause them to turn brown but they will still be delicious!
- 1 cup coconut flakes or shredded unsweetened coconut find here

Instructions

1. Place all ingredients except for the coconut and apricots in a food processor and process until a ball forms, about 2-3 minutes.

2. Pulse in apricots and coconut to chop and mix. Keep a hand on your food processor as the dense dough can cause it to 'walk' on the countertop.

3. Carefully remove blade, and then scoop dough onto parchment paper to roll out. Gently pat into a rectangle shape.

4. Roll to desired thickness (I like a little less than 1/2-inch) between two sheets of parchment paper.

5. Remove top sheet of parchment paper and flip onto a dehydrator tray.

6. Dry the whole sheet of protein bars for 6-12 hours or overnight on high, until no longer tacky. You can skip this step and go straight to cutting into bars, but it's easier to cut into even bars after drying for a little while.

7. After no longer tacky, allow sheet of dough to cool for 30 minutes to firm it up. Then flip onto a large cutting board and cut into 10 even rectangles and return to dehydrator tray. If your knife is sticking, get your knife wet and then try again.

8. Dehydrate for another 4 hours or overnight, depending on how hard you want your bars to be (longer drying time yields more firm protein bars). Bars will firm up again when they cool.

9. Store in an airtight container in the fridge for up to 1 month. These will hold up fine at room temperature for camping, hiking, etc.

Greens and Bacon Sunshine Frittata: Easy & Delicious

Prep Time: 15 Minutes

Cook Time: 20 Minutes

Total Time: 35 Minutes

Servings: 4

Calories: 344 Kcal

Ingredients

- 2 slices bacon cut into 1/2 inch slices
- 1 onion chopped
- 6 mushrooms sliced
- 4 cups loosely packed greens
- 12 eggs
- 1/4 cup coconut milk cream, or yogurt
- 1/4 teaspoon freshly ground black pepper
- 1/4 teaspoon turmeric
- 1/2 cup cheese shredded (optional)

Instructions

1. In a large cast iron skillet over medium heat, sautee bacon for 5 minutes, or until it starts to release the grease. Add in mushrooms and onion and continue to

sautee until bacon is crisp and onions are translucent. Dump in greens, and stir until wilted, about 3 more minutes.

2. Preheat oven to 375* F

3. Gently mix eggs with coconut milk, pepper and turmeric. Pour over spinach mixture and put the whole pan in the oven. Remove from oven when center of the fritatta is set and has puffed up a bit, about 20 minutes.

4. Top with cheese and return to the oven for 5 minutes, or until melted.

5. Slice into wedges and enjoy!

Homemade "No Weird Stuff" Breakfast Sausage

Prep Time: 15 Minutes

Cook Time: 15 Minutes

Total Time: 30 Minutes

Servings: 24 Patties

Calories: 172 Kcal

Ingredients

- 3 pounds ground pork beef, chicken, turkey, or a combination

- 3 teaspoon salt trouble getting your potassium? Use half lite-salt
- 1-1/2 teaspoon dried parsley
- 1 teaspoon rubbed dried sage
- 1 teaspoon ground black pepper
- 1/2 teaspoon fennel seeds
- 1/2 teaspoon crushed red pepper
- 1 teaspoon ground coriander
- 1/4 cup Bacon fat for frying

Instructions

1. In a medium mixing bowl, mix meat and all seasonings.

2. Optional: cover and chill over night to allow all the flavors to meld. This step isn't essential, but really helps the flavors to combine.

3. Heat a skillet or griddle over medium heat and grease with bacon fat or other cooking fat. Once hot, form meat mixture into patties and fry until no longer pink in the center if eating immediately, or still slightly pink if storing to reheat later.

4. For crumbled sausage, brown, breaking up chunks with a spatula. and then drain before storing.

To Store:

1. Freeze sausage patties flat on a large metal cookie sheet, then transfer to a zip-top bag or freezer container once frozen (about 6 hours). This is called flash freezing and helps prevent the sausage patties from sticking together when they are frozen.

2. Freeze browned crumbled sausage in desired portion amounts (1-1/2 cups is a good amount) in freezer bags or freezer-proof containers.

3. Use within 6 months if frozen, 7 days if refrigerated.

Pumpkin-Cranberry Low Carb Muffins

Prep Time: 10 Minutes

Cook Time: 25 Minutes

Total Time: 35 Minutes

Servings: 12 Servings

Calories: 181 Kcal

Ingredients

- 2 cups almond flour

- 2 tablespoons coconut flour
- 1-1/2 teaspoon baking powder GAPS: Omit, the eggs will provide leavening
- 1/2 teaspoon sea salt
- 1 teaspoon cinnamon
- dash nutmeg just a little
- 1/2 teaspoon monkfruit sweetener or the equivalent of 1/3 cup sugar - GAPS use 1/3 cup honey, decreasing the almond milk if the batter gets too runny
- 3/4 cup pumpkin puree
- 1/3 cup almond milk unsweetened
- 1/3 cup butter melted
- 3 eggs
- 1 cup cranberries

Instructions

1. Preheat oven to 375* F and, if using, put muffin liners in the muffin pan . Spray with avocado oil cooking spray, or melt a little butter or coconut oil into each liner to grease.

2. In a medium mixing bowl, use a fork or whisk to combine almond flour, coconut flour, baking powder if

using, sea salt, cinnamon, nutmeg, and monkfruit sweetener if using. Make sure all clumps of coconut flour are mixed up and the mixture is well combined.

3. In the same bowl, add the pumpkin puree, almond milk, melted butter, and 3 eggs. Stir to combine gently, making sure there are no dry pockets. Fold in cranberries.

4. Spoon into muffin cups, filling nearly full and smoothing out the top of the muffins gently to prevent peaks from burning. Bake for 25 minutes, checking for doneness (a toothpick inserted in a large center muffin should come out clean). Allow to cool slightly in the pan, then remove.

5. Top with butter if desired. These muffins are best warm, so reheating in a toaster oven the next day is recommended.

Greens and Bacon Sunshine Frittata

Prep Time: 15 Minutes

Cook Time: 20 Minutes

Total Time: 35 Minutes

Servings: 4

Calories: 344 Kcal

Ingredients

- 2 slices bacon cut into 1/2 inch slices
- 1 onion chopped
- 6 mushrooms sliced
- 4 cups loosely packed greens
- 12 eggs
- 1/4 cup coconut milk cream, or yogurt
- 1/4 teaspoon freshly ground black pepper
- 1/4 teaspoon turmeric
- 1/2 cup cheese shredded (optional)

Instructions

1. In a large cast iron skillet over medium heat, sautee bacon for 5 minutes, or until it starts to release the grease. Add in mushrooms and onion and continue to sautee until bacon is crisp and onions are translucent.

Dump in greens, and stir until wilted, about 3 more minutes.

2. Preheat oven to 375* F

3. Gently mix eggs with coconut milk, pepper and turmeric. Pour over spinach mixture and put the whole pan in the oven. Remove from oven when center of the fritatta is set and has puffed up a bit, about 20 minutes.

4. Top with cheese and return to the oven for 5 minutes, or until melted.

5. Slice into wedges and enjoy!

Keto Hazelnut Sandwich Bread

Prep Time: 20 Minutes

Cook Time: 30 Minutes

Total Time: 50 Minutes

Servings: 10 Slices

Calories: 167 Kcal

Ingredients
- 6 eggs separated
- 1/8 teaspoon cream of tartar

- 4 tablespoons melted butter ghee, or coconut oil (add 1/4 teaspoon salt if using coconut oil)
- 1-1/2 cups hazelnut flour find here
- 2 packets stevia or equivalent of another no-carb sweetener
- 1/2 teaspoon sea salt
- Extra hazelnut flour to sprinkle the top of the loaf optional

Instructions

1. Preheat oven to 375*F and prepare a loaf pan by greasing well with coconut oil, or (my preferred method) lining with parchment paper and then greasing that.
2. Whip the egg whites and cream of tartar (I like to use a whip attachment in a stand mixer) until stiff peaks form.
3. Mix the egg yolks, melted butter, hazelnut flour, stevia, and sea salt in a separate bowl until well combined. If it is too thick to mix well, add a little bit of the egg white (before whipping) to it until you can easily mix it.

4. Once the egg whites are fluffy, throughly but quickly and gently mix in the egg yolk mixture. You want the bread batter to be completely mixed through, but over mixing will cause the air pockets to deflate and your bread won't be as tall.

5. Pour batter into prepared loaf pan and smooth with a spatula. Batter should come up to about 1 inch below the top of the loaf pan; if there is extra, bake in a small custard cup or muffin pan. Sprinkle the top if desired with extra flour. We just sprinkle the top with flour to give it a more 'bread like' appearance.

6. Bake for 25-35 minutes, or until a knife inserted into the center of the loaf comes out clean. Allow to cool for 5 minutes in the pan, then remove from the pan and remove parchment paper and allow to cool completely on a metal cooling rack before slicing into 10 slices.

Irresistible Keto Nutella Muffins

Prep Time: 20 Minutes

Cook Time: 20 Minutes

Total Time: 40 Minutes

Servings: 10

Calories: 208 Kcal

Ingredients

- 6 eggs seperated
- 1/8 teaspoon cream of tartaroptional
- 1-1/2 cups hazelnut flour find here
- 4 tablespoons melted coconut oilghee, or MCT oil
- 1/4 teaspoon sea salt
- 4 packets stevia or 1/8 teaspoon pure monkfruit
- 1/4 cup cocoa powder
- 1/4 cup mini dark chocolate chips

Instructions

1. Preheat oven to 375* F, line a muffin pan with parchment muffin linersand spray with cooking spray or add a few drops of melted coconut oil to each muffin liner.

2. With a mixer, whip egg whites with cream of tartar until stiff peaks form. (you can skip this step but they won't rise as tall)

3. In a separate bowl mix the egg yolks, hazelnut flour, coconut oil or other fat, sea salt, stevia, cocoa powder, and dark chocolate chips.

4. Once the egg whites are firm, mix in hazelnut flour mixture briefly, but until well-combined. Do not over mix as this will deflate the eggs.

5. Distribute evenly over 10 muffin cups (depending on how large your eggs are, this may take up 9-12)

6. Bake for 20 minutes, or until a toothpick inserted in the center of a muffin comes out clean.

Lunch

Grain Free Bell Pepper And Seed Crackers

Ingredients

- 1 1/2 cups sunflower seed kernels (I used soaked and dehydrated seeds , but toasted seeds will also work well)
- 2 roasted red, orange or yellow bell peppers*
- 1/2 teaspoon dried Italian seasoning
- 1/2 teaspoon Celtic sea salt
- 1 cup shredded Pecorino Romano cheese

Instructions

1. Preheat oven to 170ºF and adjust rack to middle position. Place sunflower seeds in the bowl of a food processor. Process until finely ground. Add bell peppers, Italian seasoning, sea salt and cheese. Process until smooth.

2. Line a large baking sheet with parchment paper. Spoon mixture onto baking sheet and spread using an offset spatula until it's about 1/8" thick. Dehydrate in the oven overnight (about 7-10 hours depending on

how much humidity is in your area) until crisp. Cool to room temperature. Break apart into large crackers and store in an airtight container for up to 2 weeks.

3. *To roast the peppers: Preheat the broiler. Place the whole peppers on a baking sheet and put under the broiler. Cook until the skins are just turning black. Using a pair of tongs, turn the peppers so the black skin is facing down. Repeat until all sides of the pepper are turning black. Place peppers in a deep bowl and cover the bowl tightly with plastic wrap. Let the peppers sit for 10 minutes (the steam will loosen the skins). When the peppers are cool enough to handle, peel the skin off and remove the seeds inside the pepper.

Grain-Free Graham Crackers With Honey-Vanilla Marshmallows

Ingredients
- For the crackers:
- 2 cups almond flour
- 1/4 cup coconut flour
- 3/4 teaspoon gelatin

- 2 tablespoons honey
- 3/4 teaspoon aluminum-free baking powder
- 1/2 teaspoon baking soda
- 1/2 teaspoon coarse sea salt
- 1/8 teaspoon ground cinnamon
- 6 tablespoons cold unsalted butter, cut into 1/4-inch cubes
- 1/4 cup molasses
- 3 tablespoons whole milk or coconut milk
- 1/2 teaspoon vanilla extract
- For the Marshmallows:
- 3 tablespoons unflavored gelatin
- 2 cups honey (I prefer a light honey like clover)
- 1 vanilla bean, split, with seeds scraped out
- 1/4 teaspoon Celtic sea salt

Instructions

1. Preheat the oven to 350° F and adjust rack to middle position. Place flours, gelatin, honey, baking powder, baking soda, salt and cinnamon into the bowl of a food processor and pulse 4 times to combine. Add the butter and pulse 7 times until the mixture resembles cornmeal.

Add the molasses, milk and vanilla extract to the dough and process until the dough forms a ball. The dough will be very tacky. Pour the dough out onto a large piece of parchment paper (a piece large enough to cover a large baking sheet).

2. Dust the top of the dough with a little coconut flour. Using a rolling pin, roll the dough out until it's a rectangle about 14 x 11 inches and about 1/8-inch thick. Using a knife or rolling pizza cutter, divide it into 2 x 2-inch square pieces. There will be small pieces of excess on the sides. Using a fork, poke holes in the top of the dough. Place the baking pan with the dough in the oven and bake for 18-20 minutes or until the edges just start to darken. Remove from the oven and cool completely. Once completely cool, break into individual crackers. Store in an airtight container. The crackers will keep for 1 week.

3. For the Marshmallows: Sprinkle gelatin over 1/2 cup water in the bowl of a standing mixer with a whisk attached. Set aside for 5 minutes so the gelatin can soften and bloom. Lightly oil a 13 x 9-inch baking dish.

4. Whisk together honey and salt in a medium saucepan over medium heat. Add vanilla bean and vanilla seeds. Gently simmer until syrup reaches 240°F. With mixer on medium speed, very slowly add honey to gelatin and water in mixing bowl (it should take about 1 1/2 minutes to add all of the honey mixture). Turn mixer on high for 10 minutes until liquid has doubled and becomes light and fluffy. Pour into the oiled baking dish and let sit at room temperature overnight, uncovered.

5. The next day, flip the marshmallows onto a greased cutting board. Cut marshmallows using a knife dipped in hot water, to prevent sticking (I also oiled my hands when handling the marshmallows to prevent sticking).

Granola Bars

Ingredients

For the bars:
- 1 1/2 cups chopped almonds (dehydrated or toasted)
- 1 1/2 cups chopped cashews (dehydrated or toasted)
- 1 cup shredded unsweetened coconut

- 1 1/2 cups seeds (I used dehydrated pumpkin and sunflower seeds)
- 3 tablespoons coconut oil (or unsalted butter), melted
- 2/3 cup light honey
- 1 tablespoon vanilla extract
- 1/4 teaspoon Celtic sea salt

Instructions

1. Preheat oven to 300ºF and adjust rack to middle position. Line an 11 x 7-inch baking pan with parchment paper so the sides of paper overhang.

2. Place the almonds, cashews, coconut and seeds in a large mixing bowl. Heat oil, honey and salt in a small saucepan over medium heat. Bring to a simmer. Stir in the vanilla and pour mixture over nut mixture. Fold until incorporated. Pour mixture into the baking dish and press into the bottom of the pan. Bake for 30 minutes. Cool completely before cutting (this step is very important. If you cut while they are warm, they will fall apart). Holding onto the parchment, gently lift the bars out of the pan and place on a cutting board. Using a

large knife, cut granola into bars. Keep in an airtight container for 10 days.

3. Dehydration Method (If you took the time to soak and dehydrate your nuts and seeds then you might want to use this option to bake the bars):?Follow instructions above and dehydrate at 170ºF (or as low as your oven will go) for about 7-8 hours, until the outer edges are just slightly golden brown. Cool completely before cutting.

A few tips:

4. To ensure the granola cuts into clean uniform bars, I usually start in the middle and cut with a large chefs knife. You can also put the granola bars in the refrigerator after baking for 30 minutes to ensure the honey (the glue that binds the bars together) hardens to make cutting easier (this step can be helpful if you live in a humid climate).

Coconut Cake With Lemon Curd, Strawberries and Whipped Cream

Ingredients

For the Cake Batter:

- 1 cup coconut flour
- 1/2 teaspoon Celtic sea salt
- 8 large eggs
- 1 teaspoon baking soda
- 1/2 cup plain whole yogurt (or a coconut yogurt)
- 6 tablespoons unsalted butter or coconut oil , melted
- 1/2 cup honey (I used clover)
- 1 tablespoon vanilla extract

For the Lemon Curd:

- 8 tablespoons unsalted butter or 6 tablespoons coconut oil
- 1/2 cup honey
- 4 large eggs
- 3 large egg yolks
- 1/4 cup lemon zest (make sure the lemons are organic)

- 1/2 cup freshly squeezed lemon juice (about 6-8 lemons)
- 1/8 teaspoon Celtic sea salt
- 2 cups heavy cream or coconut milk, whipped
- 2 cups strawberries, tops removed, cut in half

Instructions

1. Preheat oven to 350ºF and adjust rack to middle position. Butter a 9" round cake pan and dust with coconut flour (this will ensure the cake doesn't stick). Place all cake ingredients in the bowl of a food processor and blend until smooth. Pour batter into the buttered cake pan and bake for 40-45 minutes, or until just turning golden brown on top and a cake tester inserted in the middle of the cake comes out clean. Cool for ten minutes, then run a knife around the edges and invert onto a cake platter. Cool completely.

2. Melt butter in a double boiler set over medium heat. Whisk together honey, eggs, yolks, zest, juice and salt in a large measuring cup. Slowly, while constantly whisking, pour in egg mixture and continue to whisk for 6-8 minutes until thick like pudding. Pour curd through

a fine mesh sieve over a medium bowl, cover and chill in the refrigerator for 2 hours or until cold.

To assemble:

3. Cut cake in half. Spoon half of curd mixture on top of bottom cake layer and spread evenly. Spoon half of whipped cream on top of curd and spread evenly. Top with 1 cup berries. Place second cake layer on top and repeat with curd, cream and berries, Serve.

Homemade Coconut Almond Joy Candy Bars

Ingredients

For the bars:

- 2 cups unsweetened coconut
- 1/3 cup maple syrup
- 12 whole almonds
- 6 ounces dark chocolate , melted
- 1 tablespoon virgin coconut oil

Instructions

1. Place coconut and maple syrup in the bowl of a food processor. Process for 2 minutes, until coconut is very moist and clumps together when squeezed between

your fingers. Place a cooling rack on top of a large baking sheet. Using your hands, take about 1 1/2 tablespoons of the coconut mixture and form it into an oval. Place on the cooling rack. Repeat with remaining coconut. Place an almond on top of each coconut mound. Whisk together the chocolate and coconut oil until smooth. Using a large spoon, spoon about a tablespoon of chocolate over each coconut/almond mound. Refrigerate for 10 minutes until firm. Serve.

Grain Free Bell Pepper and Seed

Ingredients

- 1 1/2 cups sunflower seed kernels (I used soaked and dehydrated seeds , but toasted seeds will also work well)
- 2 roasted red, orange or yellow bell peppers*
- 1/2 teaspoon dried Italian seasoning
- 1/2 teaspoon Celtic sea salt
- 1 cup shredded Pecorino Romano

Instructions

1. Preheat oven to 170ºF and adjust rack to middle position. Place sunflower seeds in the bowl of a food processor. Process until finely ground. Add bell peppers, Italian seasoning, sea salt and cheese. Process until smooth.

2. Line a large baking sheet with parchment paper. Spoon mixture onto baking sheet and spread using an offset spatula until it's about 1/8" thick. Dehydrate in the oven overnight (about 7-10 hours depending on how much humidity is in your area) until crisp. Cool to room temperature. Break apart into large crackers and store in an airtight container for up to 2 weeks.

3. *To roast the peppers:Preheat the broiler. Place the whole peppers on a baking sheet and put under the broiler. Cook until the skins are just turning black. Using a pair of tongs, turn the peppers so the black skin is facing down. Repeat until all sides of the pepper are turning black. Place peppers in a deep bowl and cover the bowl tightly with plastic wrap. Let the peppers sit for 10 minutes (the steam will loosen the skins). When

the peppers are cool enough to handle, peel the skin off and remove the seeds inside the pepper.

Creamy Chicken, Tomato and Vegetable Soup

Serves 6

Ingredients

- 4 tablespoons unsalted butter (or 3 tablespoons coconut oil for a dairy-free option)
- 4 large carrots, chopped
- 1 large leek, chopped
- 2 ribs celery, chopped
- 4 cloves garlic, minced
- 8 ounces mushrooms, sliced
- 2 teaspoons Celtic sea salt, divided
- 2 teaspoons dried Italian seasoning
- 4 cups chicken stock or meat stock
- 3 boneless, skinless chicken breasts
- 1 (24-ounce) jar crushed tomatoes
- 1/2 cup heavy cream (or canned coconut milk for a dairy-free alternative)

Instructions

1. Melt butter in a large pot . Add carrots, leek, celery and garlic. Stir. Cover pot and reduce heat to low. Cook for 30 minutes. Add mushrooms and 1 teaspoon sea salt to pot. Stir and cook for 10 minutes. Stir in Italian seasoning and cook for 1 minute. Add stock, chicken, tomatoes and remaining 1 teaspoon salt. Bring to a simmer and cook until chicken is cooked through, about 10 minutes. Remove chicken from pot, chop into bite-size pieces and add back to the soup. Pour in cream and season to taste. Serve.

Tortilla Soup Recipe

Prep Time: 15 min
Cook Time: 30 min
Total Time: 45 min
Ingredients

For the soup:

- 5 cloves garlic, crushed with skins on
- 6 springs fresh oregano
- 6 sprigs of cilantro, plus 1/2 cup roughly chopped
- 8 cups chicken stock

- 2 pounds bone-in chicken breasts or 1 small 3-4 pound chicken

For the Toppings:

- 3 cups Siete tortilla chips
- 1 avocado, cubed
- 2 tomatoes, cut into bite-size chunks
- 1 lime, cut into quarters
- 1/2 cup sour cream
- 1/2 cup shredded cheddar cheese

Instructions

1. Place the garlic cloves in a large dutch oven over medium-high heat. Cook, stirring frequently until garlic begins to darken, about 2-2 1/2 minutes. Remove the pot from the heat and let it cool for about 30 seconds and then add the chicken stock, oregano, cilantro, and chicken to the garlic. Place pot back on heat and bring to a boil and then reduce to a simmer. Simmer for about 30 minutes. When chicken is cooked through, remove the chicken from the broth mixture and set aside. With slotted spoon, strain out the rest of the

garlic and herbs. Shred the chicken with a fork and then add back to the soup. Add salt and pepper if needed.

2. To serve, crumble a handful of tortilla chips into individual bowls and then ladle the broth over. Serve with cilantro, avocado, tomatoes, lime, cheese, and sour cream.

Blueberry

Ingredients

For the batter:

- 6 large eggs
- 1/3 cup heavy cream or coconut milk
- 1/4 cup honey
- 1 teaspoon vanilla
- 1 stick (8 tablespoons) unsalted butter, melted
- 3/4 cup plus 2 tablespoons coconut flour
- 2 teaspoons baking powder*
- 1 teaspoon baking soda
- 3/4 teaspoon Celtic sea salt
- 1/2 cup applesauce
- 1 1/2 cups blueberries, frozen (no need to thaw them)

Instructions

1. Preheat oven to 375ºF and adjust rack to middle position. Line muffin pan with muffin liners. Whisk eggs, cream, honey, vanilla and butter in a large mixing bowl. Sift coconut flour, baking powder, baking soda, and salt over a medium bowl. Add wet ingredients to dry ingredients and whisk until no lumps remain. Fold in applesauce and then fold in blueberries. Spoon batter into muffin cups. Bake for 18 minutes, or until lightly brown on top. Store muffins in an airtight container for 3 days.

Pumpkin Muffins With Chocolate Chips

Ingredients

For the Batter:

- 6 large eggs
- 1/3 cup heavy
- 1/4 cup plus 2 tablespoons coconut sugar or maple sugar
- 1 teaspoon vanilla extract

- 8 tablespoons unsalted butter, melted (or coconut oil for dairy-free)
- 3/4 cup coconut flour
- 2 teaspoons grain-free baking powder (see above)
- 1 teaspoon baking soda
- 3/4 teaspoon Celtic sea salt
- 1 cup cooked and pureed pumpkin
- 5 ounces organic mini chocolate chips, or chopped bittersweet chocolate

Instructions

1. Preheat oven to 400 degrees F and adjust rack to middle position. Line muffin pan with muffin liners. Whisk eggs, cream (or coconut milk), coconut sugar, vanilla and butter in a large mixing bowl. Sift coconut flour, baking powder, baking soda, and salt over a medium mixing bowl. Add dry ingredients to wet and whisk until no lumps remain. Fold in pumpkin and chocolate. Spoon batter into muffin cups. Bake for 15 minutes, until golden brown on top. Cool. Store muffins in an airtight container for 3 days.

Main Dishes

Tritip, Baked

Prep Time: 5 Minutes

Cook Time: 35 Minutes

Resting Time: 10 Minutes

Servings: 6

Calories: 373 Kcal

Ingredients

• 3 pound tritip roast

• 1 tablespoon tallow, ghee, or bacon grease softened, more if your tritip has been trimmed of most fat.

• 1/2 teaspoon sea salt to taste

Instructions

1. Preheat a skillet to medium-high heat. Preheat oven to 350*

2. Cover tritip with sea salt and softened fat, on both sides. Allow to rest for 5 minutes as the skillet completely preheats.

3. Placing fat-cap down, sear the tritip in the skillet for 3-4 minutes, or until golden.

4. Flip onto a parchment-covered baking dish. Bake, with seared fat-side up for 10 minutes per pound, or 25 minutes for a 2-1/2 pound tritip; 30 minutes for a 3-pound tritip.

5. After baking, allow to rest for 10 minutes before slicing across the grain of the meat and serving.

Parmesan-Pork Meatballs

Ingredients

- 2 pounds ground pork
- 1 cup shredded parmesan cheese
- 2 eggs optional
- 1 teaspoon sea salt

Instructions

1. Mix together the ground pork, parmesan cheese, and optional eggs. The cheese has plenty of salt, but you may want to cook a bit of the meat mixture in a pan on the stove and adjust the salt if needed - add 1 teaspoon of sea salt at a time until you get the saltiness that you like.

2. Preheat broiler to high. Raise rack to the second slot down from the top in the oven. Line a metal baking tray with shallow sides (like a jelly roll pan) with parchment paper.

3. As the oven heats, roll meatballs into desired size (I like smaller acorn-sized meatballand place on the lined baking sheet; touching but not overlapping. Make sure your meatballs are all the same size so that they cook evenly.

4. Once preheated, broil the meatballs for 5 minutes, or until tops start to darken. If you are freezing the meatballs, remove them now and cool, then transfer to a freezer bag. Reheat/finish cooking from thawed, 350* for 20 minutes or until cooked through.

5. Move meatballs to the middle of the oven and turn the oven to 'bake' and 350* and bake for an additional 15-20 minutes, depending on how big your meatballs are.

6. To check doneness, cut meatball in half. Slight pink in the middle is okay, as they will continue cooking as they cool.

7. Serve your meatballs, topping with more cheese or cream sauce as desired.

Bacon Cheeseburger Casserole

Prep Time: 30 Minutes

Cook Time: 20 Minutes

Servings: 6 Servings

Calories: 574 Kcal

Ingredients

- 4 slices bacon
- 1/2 pound mushrooms sliced, optional
- 1 small onion diced, optional
- 2 lbs ground beef ground elk or part venison can also be used. Pictured recipe uses elk, which cooks up similarly to beef.
- 1/4 cup no-sugar ketchup optional
- 2 tablespoons mustard optional
- 1/2 teaspoon sea salt
- 3 eggs
- 1-1/2 cups shredded cheddar cheese
- 1/2 cup sour cream optional

Instructions

1. In a large skillet over medium heat cook bacon until still soft, but mostly cooked. Leave the bacon grease in the skillet and stir in optional onions and/or mushrooms if using until soft. Next brown beef in the bacon fat, with the optional mushrooms/onions if using.

2. Once beef is browned, mix in the optional ketchup and mustard, sea salt, and eggs.

3. Preheat oven to 400* If you're using an oven-proof skillet, you can bake the casserole right in the skillet. If not, grease a casserole dish and transfer the ground beef mixture to the casserole dish, spreading in evenly. Top with cheddar cheese. Cut the bacon into small pieces and sprinkle on top of the cheese.

4. Bake for 20 minutes, or until cheese is melted and bacon is crisp. Allow to stand for 5 minutes before serving with sour cream if desired.

Garlic-Mushroom Chicken With Parmesan And Bacon

Prep Time: 30 Minutes

Cook Time: 30 Minutes

Total Time: 1 Hour

Servings: 8 Chicken Thighs

Calories: 553 Kcal

Ingredients

For The Chicken:

- 1 tablespoon butter
- 8 chicken thighs preferably skin on bone out but any chicken thighs work
- 1/4 teaspoon sea salt
- pinch freshly ground black pepper

For The Garlic Cream Sauce:

- 8 cloves garlic crushed
- 8 ounces bacon chopped into 1/2-inch pieces
- 16 ounces baby portabello mushrooms
- 1 cup heavy cream GAPS use 24-hour yogurt
- 4 ounces parmesan grated (about 3/4 cup grated)
- salt to taste

- 1 tablespoon parsley

Instructions

Make The Chicken:

1. Preheat oven to 400* F. In a large skillet, melt butter over medium-high heat. Careful, it's hot! (duh. but I totally burned myself the first time I made this.) Once skillet is pre-heated, sear the chicken for 3-4 minutes on each side, until starting to turn golden brown. You will probably have to do this in batches.

2. Once seared, place skin-side up in a 9×13" or similarly sized casserole dish. Once all the chicken is in the dish, sprinkle with sea salt and bake for 20 minutes if boneless, or 30 minutes for bone-in.

Make The Cream Sauce:

1. As the chicken bakes, using the same pan that you used to sear the chicken (without draining), add crushed garlic and sautee until turning fragrant and starting to brown, just a minute or two.

2. Add chopped bacon to the garlic and cook, stirring every minute or two, until bacon starts to crisp but is still slightly soft. While the bacon cooks, slice your

mushrooms. Use a slotted spoon to remove bacon once desired doneness.

3. Once bacon is removed, add in mushrooms and cook in the bacon grease until soft. Once soft, add in cream and give the mushrooms a stir. By now the chicken should be nearly done, if not, just remove the cream and mushrooms from the heat.

4. Once chicken is done pour the cream/mushrooms over the chicken, sprinkle with parmesan, then parsley, then reserved bacon. Return to the oven for 10 minutes to allow all the flavors to combine.

Crackslaw

Prep Time: 5 Minutes
Cook Time: 20 Minutes
Total Time: 25 Minutes
Servings: 4 Servings
Calories: 440 Kcal

Ingredients
- 2 tablespoons coconut oil or bacon grease

- 1/2 teaspoon ground ginger or 1 tablespoon fresh grated
- 3 cloves garlic crushed
- 2 pounds ground turkey or pork, chicken, or beef, or a combination
- 2 tablespoons soy sauce or 3 tablespoons coconut aminos
- 1 teaspoon fish sauce Red Boat brand, optional
- 1 pound coleslaw mix or half a green cabbage, shredded
- 5 green onions just the white and light green prats
- Optional: Sprinkle of sesame seedstoasted, a couple tablespoons
- Optional: sesame oil to drizzle on top
- 1/4 cup Chili Lime Dressing Recipe linked

Instructions

1. In a large skillet over medium-high heat, melt coconut oil or bacon grease.

2. Once fat is melted, add garlic and ginger and sauté for a minute, until garlic starts releasing its aroma. Add

in turkey, breaking it up to brown it. Reduce heat to medium if needed and brown turkey.

3. As the turkey browns, thinly slice the green onions, just the white and light green parts, and set aside.

4. Once turkey is browned, add in coleslaw mix or green cabbage and soy sauce or coconut aminos and optional fish sauce.

5. Saute the cabbage in with the turkey until it is wilted.

6. Serve from the pan, and top each serving with: Chili Lime Dressing, additional hot sauce if desired, sliced green onions, and a sprinkle of sesame seeds.

Paleo Chicken Enchilada Bowls In Spaghetti Squash

Prep Time: 20 Minutes
Cook Time: 45 Minutes
Total Time: 1 Hour 5 Minutes
Servings: 4 People
Calories: 263 Kcal

Ingredients
- 2 medium spaghetti squash

- 1 tablespoon coconut oil
- 1 pound boneless chicken thighs or breasts
- 6 oz tomato paste
- 1 teaspoon sea salt
- 1/2 teaspoon cayenne
- 1/2 teaspoon cumin
- 1 teaspoon smoked paprika
- 1 teaspoon dried oregano
- 1/2 onion diced
- 1-1/2 cups chicken stock

Instructions

1. Preheat oven to 350*. Cut spaghetti squash in half. Scoop out pulp and seeds, leaving the 1-2 inches of rind in the squash. Place cut-side down on a roasting pan or two. Fill pans with 1 inch of filtered water and place in the oven for 45 minutes.

2. In a large sauce pan, melt coconut oil over medium heat. As the oil is melting, cut up chicken into bite-sized pieces. Add the chicken all at once, and stir occasionally.

3. As you are stirring the chicken, make the enchilada sauce by mixing the tomato paste, spices, and onion in a small bowl with a fork. Gradually add chicken stock to thin the mixture.

4. Once the chicken has been browned, reduce heat to medium-low and add the enchilada sauce. Cover. Allow to simmer, covered, stirring every 10 minutes or so, until the squash is done.

5. Once the squash is done, remove from heat and allow it to cool for 5 minutes. Remove the chicken-enchilada sauce mixture from the heat as well.

6. Use a fork to separate all the spaghetti strings of each squash half, leaving the squash in the bowl for serving. Top with the chicken enchilada mixture and toppings of choice. Enjoy hot!

Spaghetti Squash

Prep Time: 10 Minutes

Cook Time: 10 Minutes

Cooling Time: 15 Minutes

Total Time: 20 Minutes

Servings: 6 Cups

Calories: 22 Kcal

Ingredients

- 1 Spaghetti Squash 4-5 lbs

Instructions

1. Cut spaghetti squash in half crosswise (be careful!) using a large knife. Use a large spoon to scrape the strings and seeds, reserving if desired for roasted squash seeds.
2. Cook your spaghetti squash using your method of choice below.
3. Squash is done when it slightly gives and can be pierced with a fork, but is not mushy. Mushy squash still tastes good, but it won't have the defined spaghetti strands that are so unique. It will continue to cook a bit as it cools.

Instant Pot:

1. Fill pot with 2 cups of water (use the lines on the side of your pot), place a trivet or steamer basket in, and place squash cut-side down on the trivet or steamer basket in the Instant Pot.

2. Depending on the shape of your squash and size of your Instant Pot, you may need to do two batches to get the whole squash cooked - no worries, this is a very fast method and you'll have them both done in no time! If you can fit them both in and still close the lid, you can do both halves at once.

3. Close the lid, and set the vent to seal. Set the Instant Pot to Manual - 8 minutes* and allow to come to pressure. Naturally let the pressure come down for 5 minutes after it is done cooking, and then use quick release to release the rest of the pressure. Set squash aside to cool until comfortable to touch (15 minutes) before using a fork to scrape out the spaghetti strands.

4. If necessary, repeat with the other squash half.

* *Instant Pots can take some getting used to. If your spaghetti squash is too soft after the 8 minutes on pressure and 5 minutes natural pressure release, yours might run a little hot. In contrast, if it is still firm, even after the 15 minutes of cooling, it might run a bit low and you'll want to add a minute or two to the cooking time for most recipes.

Finally, if your squash is barely cooked at all, you probably need to replace the silicone ring around the lid.

This modern gadget can save oodles of time in the kitchen, but it does take some patience to get it to work how we want it to.

Slow Cooker:

1. First, check to make sure your squash fits in the slow cooker! You can cut it into large 'rings' instead of just in half if necessary to make it fit. By keeping it cut crosswise, we get longer squash 'noodles' so try to avoid cutting it lengthwise.

2. Pour 1 cup of water into the bottom of a slow cooker. Place squash cut-side down in the slow cooker and cook on low for 4-5 hours or high for 2 hours.

3. Open lid and turn off slow cooker and allow squash to cool until comfortable to touch (15 minutes) before using a fork to scrape out the spaghetti strands.

Oven Roasted:

1. Preheat oven to 400* F.

2. Optionally, brush squash ends (cut side) with olive oil, melted butter, or coconut oil. Place cut-side down in a casserole dish or baking sheet *with sides* to contain juices. Add 1 cup of water.

3. Place squash in the oven (it's okay if it hasn't completely preheated yet) and bake for 45 minutes.

4. Remove from the oven and allow squash to cool until comfortable to touch (15 minutes) before using a fork to scrape out the spaghetti strands.

Keto Broccoli Chicken Casserole

Prep Time: 25 Minutes

Cook Time: 35 Minutes

Total Time: 55 Minutes

Servings: 6 Servings

Calories: 576 Kcal

Ingredients

- 1 tablespoon butter
- 2 pounds boneless skinless chicken thighs
- 1 tablespoon apple cider vinegar or 1/4 cup white wine
- 2 pounds broccoli or broccoli/cauliflower combination
- 8 ounces cream cheese
- 8 ounces cheddar cheese grated
- 1 tablespoon dried onion
- 1/2 pinch nutmeg just a tiny bit- less than 1/8 tsp
- 1/4 teaspoon black pepper
- 1/4 teaspoon sea salt
- 1/4 cup grated parmesan cheeseoptional
- 1 cup pork rinds crushed, optional
- Cooking spray or more butter to grease casserole dish

Instructions

1. Preheat oven to 375*

2. In a large skillet, melt butter over medium high heat. Once butter is melted, add chicken and brown for 3-4 minutes on each side. Remove chicken and set aside to cool. Add apple cider vinegar or white wine to pan and deglaze, scraping off the browned bits with a wooden spoon. Reduce heat to medium low and add cream cheese, cheddar cheese, dried onion, nutmeg, black pepper, sea salt, and parmesan cheese.

3. Stir until cream cheese has softened, about 5 minutes. Remove from heat. Add in chopped broccoli or broccoli/cauliflower combination and stir. Set aside. Cut now-cooled chicken into bite-sized pieces and add to the broccoli/cheese mixture and mix in.

4. Spray a 4-quart casserole dish with cooking spray or grease with butter or coconut oil and pour in the broccoli/cheese/chicken mixture. Crush pork rinds in a bag with a rolling pin and sprinkle on top.

5. Bake for 35 minutes, or until hot all the way through. Allow to sit for 5 minutes before serving.

Homemade Fried Cheese Sticks

Prep Time: 15 Minutes

Cook Time: 30 Minutes

Total Time: 45 Minutes

Servings: 6

Calories: 267 Kcal

Ingredients

- 12 cheese sticks: Monterey Jack Cheese is recommended for the GAPS and SCD diets Mozzarella (string cheese) would work well too
- 4 eggs
- 1 cup blanched almond flour
- 1 tablespoon Italian Seasoning
- 2 cups expeller pressed coconut oil

Instructions

1. A few hours or more before put cheese sticks in the freezer. You can cut your own sticks from a large block of cheese, or purchase pre-wrapped string cheese or cheese sticks. If using string cheese, cut in half crosswise. When ready to make the fried cheese sticks, heat the oil over medium heat in as small of a sauce

pan as you can fit the cheese sticks in. Using a small pan allows the oil to be deeper.

2. In a shallow bowl or dish mix almond flour with Italian Seasoning. Lightly beat eggs in another shallow dish. Take frozen cheese sticks out and dip 1 to 3 at a time in the egg, allow egg to drip off, and then roll in the almond flour mixture until well covered. Drop into the hot oil and fry for 1-2 minutes, or until golden brown. The cheese sticks will likely float to the top of the oil at this time. Remove from oil and drain on

Salmon Patties With Green Peas

Prep Time: 15 Minutes
Cook Time: 10 Minutes
Total Time: 25 Minutes
Servings: 4
Calories: 243 Kcal

Ingredients
- Three 5-ounce cans of wild caught salmon find here
- 2 eggs

- 1/4 cup shredded coconut optional, omit one egg if not using; can also use almond meal or even almond flour (find here)
- 2-3 tablespoons ghee or coconut oil for frying

Instructions

1. Open and drain salmon by pressing cut lid on top of the salmon firmly while turning upside down over the sink.
2. Place salmon, eggs, and shredded coconut in a bowl and mix with a fork until egg is throughly distributed. This does not need to be a puree, but should be uniform.
3. Allow salmon mixture to rest (this helps the coconut to hold the mixture together) while you heat a large skillet or griddle (flat side) over medium heat.
4. Once skillet is pre-heated, add 1 tablespoon of fat and allow to melt. As the fat melts, form small patties out of the salmon, 'slider' size, or mini-burger size.
5. Once the edges start to look firm, and the top of the uncooked patty is also starting to loose its shine a little bit, - about 5 minutes of cooking- use a thin metal

spatula to carefully flip. The side that is cooked should be starting to brown.

6. Cook for another 3 minutes on the other side and then serve.

Delicious Zucchini Lasagna

Prep Time: 1 Hour

Cook Time: 45 Minutes

Total Time: 1 Hour 45 Minutes

Servings: 15

Calories: 377 Kcal

Ingredients

- 9-10 Zucchini medium-small
- 2 tablespoons avocado oil to grease skillet with
- 32 ounces tomato sauce sugar free
- 3 pounds ground beef
- 3 cloves garlic crushed
- 1/2 teaspoon freshly ground black pepper
- 1 teaspoon dried parsley
- 1 teaspoon dried basil
- 1 teaspoon sea salt

- 32 ounces ricotta cheese not allowed on GAPS, but many people tolerate it
- 16 ounces mozarella cheeseshredded (white cheddar can be used for GAPS)

Instructions

1. Heat a griddle over medium heat and grease with avocado oil.
2. Grill zucchini slices side by side, 5 minutes on each side, or until soft and becoming translucent. Set aside cooked zucchini slices and continue with batches of zucchini.
3. As you grill the zucchini slices, brown the ground beef in a large pan.
4. Mix 1/2 teaspoon sea salt and 1 clove garlic, crushed, into the ricotta cheese.
5. After the beef is browned, add the tomato sauce, 2 cloves crushed garlic, pepper, parsley, basil, and 1 teaspoon sea salt.
6. Grease three 8x8 or 10x10-inch pans with avocado oil.

7. Layer a single layer of zucchini slices in the bottom of each pan.

8. Next layer meat sauce, ricotta, zucchini, and continue as you have fillings.

9. Top with mozarella evenly, and cover with foil.

10. Put container in a freezer bag and put in the freezer.

11. To bake that day, keep covered with foil and bake at 350* for 30 minutes, then remove foil and continue cooking for 15 more minutes uncovered.

12. To thaw frozen lasagana for later, thaw overnight in the fridge, bake at 350* for 45 minutes covered, and again, 15 minutes uncovered.

Filled Summer Salad

Prep Time: 20 Minutes
Total Time: 20 Minutes
Servings: 4
Calories: 365 Kcal

Ingredients
- 3 hearts Romaine sliced across

- 1 avocado cut into slices
- 1 chicken breast coooked and cubed
- 5 hard boiled eggs sliced
- 1/2 cup shredded parmesan cheese
- 1/2 cup sunflower seeds
- Ranch Dressing
- Toss all ingredients. If you're not going to eat it all at once top each serving with dressing individually.

Instructions

1. If needed, make ranch dressing (here) and boil eggs.
2. Layer all ingredients in a large bowl, or set ingredients out on a plate so everyone can top their lettuce with the toppings they desire.
3. If you're not going to eat it all at once, top each serving with dressing individually.

Fresh Lemongrass-Ginger Grilled Pork Skewers

Prep Time: 20 Minutes
Cook Time: 10 Minutes
Total Time: 30 Minutes
Servings: 8

Calories: 408 Kcal

Ingredients

- 3-4- pound pork shoulder find here
- 2 stalks lemongrass about 4-6 inches
- 1 large shallot or half a small white onion
- 1/4 cup fish sauce this kind
- 2 tablespoons coconut aminos this kind
- 6 cloves garlic
- 1/4 cup olive oil this kind
- 1 teaspoon ground dried ginger or 1 tablespoon fresh

Instructions

1. Rinse lemongrass, and remove ends. Cut stalks into 1/2-inch or smaller pieces so that your food processor can break it up.
2. Peel ginger if using fresh and pulse with the lemongrass in the food processor.
3. Peel shallot and garlic.
4. In the food processor, place cut lemongrass stalks, peeled shallot and garlic, fish sauce, coconut aminos, olive oil, and ginger.
5. Puree to make a paste.

6. Moving to the pork roast, cut away excess fat and cut roast into approximately 1 to 1-1/2 inch cubes.

7. Once pork has been cubed, toss it with marinade to evenly coat.

8. Since the marinade is a paste, it will stick to the meat well and can be threaded onto skewers immediately.

9. Gently remove cubes of pork, keeping as much marinade on as possible, and thread onto the soaked skewers in the desired amounts.

10. Pork should be touching, but not packed tightly on the skewer. This allows all sides of the pork cube to be exposed to heat as it cooks, and the whole skewer of meat will cook evenly.

11. Rub on extra marinade to coat skewered pork - this just continues to add delicious flavor!

To Freeze: (Optional;

Allow To Sit In Marinade At Least 2 Hours If Not Freezing)

1. Using wire cutters, snip off ends of the wooden skewers and place in freezer bags. Freeze 4-6 skewers

in each bag, so you can just pull one bag at a time out of the freezer to thaw.

To Grill:

1. Thaw pork skewers that you are going to grill in the fridge overnight. If they are still icy, thaw in a cool water bath as you heat up the grill.

2. Preheat the grill to medium-high for 5-10 minutes.

3. Carefully place skewers on the grill. Try to position skewers so that the meat is over the hot spots, and the wood skewers are not over the flame too much. This will help prevent them from catching on fire.

4. Close grill and allow to cook for 3 minutes with the lid on, then remove the lid and turn as needed, browning each side.

5. Carefully watch, some kebabs will be done faster than others due to the heat pockets on the grill. Pork is done when juices run clear. As they are done, move them to the edges, or even turn off a heat element and keep the kebabs on the grill, but not over heat.

Baked Keto Cheese Taco Shells

Prep Time: 5 Minutes

Cook Time: 10 Minutes

Total Time: 15 Minutes

Ingredients

- 6 ounces white cheddar cheeseyellow cheddar is just fine too

Instructions

1. Preheat oven to 350* F
2. Line two baking sheets with parchment paper
3. Grate cheese using a cheese grater
4. Make little circular piles of cheese that are about 3" across (see picture), 3 on each baking sheet for a standard sized baking sheet. Leave lots of space between for the cheese to melt.
5. Bake for 10-12 minutes, or until edges start to turn dark and the cheese is still very melty in the middle. If you have a standard oven (not convection) rotate trays half way through to evenly cook the cheese.
6. Allow to cool on the cookie sheet for 5 minutes, the cheese will set.

7. Fill with your favorite taco fillings, and enjoy this keto-friendly taco shell!

Grain Free Low-Carb Coconut Flour Crepes

Prep Time: 15 Minutes

Cook Time: 10 Minutes

Total Time: 25 Minutes

Servings: 12

Calories: 102 Kcal

Ingredients

- 12 eggs
- 4 tablespoons fine coconut flour find here
- 1/8 teaspoon sea salt
- 6 teaspoons refined coconut oil or ghee to fry

Instructions

1. Mix all ingredients well, making sure all clumps of coconut flour are broken up. Allow to sit for a few minutes and then mix again.

2. In a skillet over medium-low heat melt 1 teaspoon of coconut oil, tilting pan to coat and allow pan to preheat well to prevent sticking.

3. Add about 2 tablespoons of batter and tilt to make a 6-inch circle.

4. Cook crepe until bubbles start to form and the middle of the pancake looks slightly cooked. Flip gently with a thin spatula and cook until the other side is golden; about 5 minutes on the first side, 2 on the second.

5. Enjoy!

Grain-Free Southern-Style Biscuits Made With Honey

Prep Time: 15 Minutes

Cook Time: 15 Minutes

Total Time: 30 Minutes

Servings: 8

Calories: 265 Kcal

Ingredients

- 2-1/2 cups blanched almond flourfind here
- 1/2 teaspoon baking soda
- 1/4 teaspoon sea salt
- 3 tablespoons unsalted butter or coconut oil, melted

- 1 tablespoon honey omit for keto or replace with 1 packet/scoop of stevia or monk fruit if desired
- 2 tablespoons coconut milk
- 2 large eggs
- ¼ teaspoon apple cider vinegar

Instructions

1. Preheat oven to 350°F. Line a baking sheet with parchment paper; set aside.
2. n a small bowl, combine almond flour, baking soda, and salt.
3. In a medium bowl, whisk together melted butter and honey until smooth. Add the coconut milk, eggs, and apple cider vinegar, whisking together until well combined.
4. Using a spoon, stir the dry mixture into the wet mixture until thoroughly combined.
5. Scoop a large spoonful of batter into your hands and gently roll into a ball about the size of an apricot; repeat until you've made
6. Place the dough balls on a parchment-lined baking sheet two inches apart and gently flatten using the

palm of your hand. (If dough is too sticky, refrigerate for about 15 minutes before rolling into balls and flattening.)

7. Bake about 15 minutes, until golden brown on top and a toothpick inserted into center comes out clean. Serve warm with a drizzle of raw honey or homemade jam.

Meatza

Prep Time: 15 Minutes

Cook Time: 30 Minutes

Total Time: 45 Minutes

Servings: 4 Servings

Calories: 838 Kcal

Ingredients

- 2 pounds ground beef
- ½ teaspoon ground black pepper
- ½ teaspoon sea salt ground
- 1 teaspoon Italian seasoning
- 1-3 cloves garlic crushed
- ½ cup tomato sauce

- 3-4 mushrooms sliced
- ½ onion diced
- 1 bell pepper sliced
- 1 tomato sliced (optional)
- 1 cup spinach shredded (optional)
- 1/3 cup olives sliced (optional)
- 2 cups Monterey Jack cheeseshredded (optional)

Instructions

1. Mix ground beef, pepper, salt, seasoning and garlic in a bowl. On a cookie sheet or in a large glass dish, pat meat into a 'pizza crust'. Top with tomato sauce and vegetables then top with cheese.

2. Bake at 400 degrees Fahrenheit for 30 minutes, or until the meat is cooked through and cheese is melted. Allow to cool for 5 minutes then slice into wedges.

3. Dairy-free: Omit cheese – eating slices of meatza is still fun anyway!

Dairy-Free Keto Baked 'Fried' Chicken Nuggets

Prep Time: 15 Minutes

Cook Time: 35 Minutes

Total Time: 50 Minutes

Servings: 4

Calories: 585 Kcal

Ingredients

• 2 pounds boneless skinless chicken thighs or tenders, nutrition calculated with thighs, cut into bite-sized pieces or thin strips

• 2 eggs

• 1.5 cups almond flour If allergic, other nut flours can be used too.

• 1 tablespoon dried parsley

• 1/2 teaspoon sea salt

• 1/2 teaspoon paprika optional

• 1/4 teaspoon freshly ground black pepper

• 2 tablespoons coconut oil to grease pan optional, use parchment if omitting

Instructions

1. Preheat oven to 375* F

2. Grease two 9x13 pans, or one cookie sheet with shallow sides OR line with parchment paper.

3. Gently mix eggs in a shallow bowl with a fork or whisk.

4. Combine almond flour, parsley, salt, paprika, and pepper in another shallow bowl. Alternative: Mix above dry ingredients in a gallon ziplock for 'shake and bake' method.

5. Dip chicken pieces in beaten eggs, in batches, and then remove and place in the almond flour mixture. When transferring from the egg to the almond flour mixture, hold the chicken above the egg bowl for a moment to allow excess to drip off.

6. Press egg-drenched chicken into almond flour mixture. Shake and bake method: Shake about 1 cup of egg-covered chicken in a gallon zip top bag (do not press out air) until evenly coated.

7. Place coated chicken on the prepared pans or cookie sheet close together but not overlapping. They can be touching in some places. Repeat the egg and almond flour steps with the remaining chicken.

8. Bake for 20-35 minutes. Lighter meat and smaller pieces will cook faster, darker meat and larger pieces will take longer to cook. Chicken is done when it feels firm and not squishy when pressed, or when cut into if it is not pink any more and juices run clear.

9. Serve while hot! Leftovers are delicious too, reheated (pan frying in a little ghee is delicious) or cold.

Keto Hazelnut Sandwich Bread

Prep Time: 20 Minutes

Cook Time: 30 Minutes

Total Time: 50 Minutes

Servings: 10 Slices

Calories: 167 Kcal

Ingredients

- 6 eggs separated
- 1/8 teaspoon cream of tartar
- 4 tablespoons melted butter ghee, or coconut oil (add 1/4 teaspoon salt if using coconut oil)
- 1-1/2 cups hazelnut flour find here

- 2 packets stevia or equivalent of another no-carb sweetener
- 1/2 teaspoon sea salt
- Extra hazelnut flour to sprinkle the top of the loaf optional

Instructions

1. Preheat oven to 375*F and prepare a loaf pan by greasing well with coconut oil, or (my preferred method) lining with parchment paper and then greasing that.
2. Whip the egg whites and cream of tartar (I like to use a whip attachment in a stand mixer) until stiff peaks form.
3. Mix the egg yolks, melted butter, hazelnut flour, stevia, and sea salt in a separate bowl until well combined. If it is too thick to mix well, add a little bit of the egg white (before whipping) to it until you can easily mix it.
4. Once the egg whites are fluffy, throughly but quickly and gently mix in the egg yolk mixture. You want the bread batter to be completely mixed through, but over

mixing will cause the air pockets to deflate and your bread won't be as tall.

5. Pour batter into prepared loaf pan and smooth with a spatula. Batter should come up to about 1 inch below the top of the loaf pan; if there is extra, bake in a small custard cup or muffin pan. Sprinkle the top if desired with extra flour. We just sprinkle the top with flour to give it a more 'bread like' appearance.

6. Bake for 25-35 minutes, or until a knife inserted into the center of the loaf comes out clean. Allow to cool for 5 minutes in the pan, then remove from the pan and remove parchment paper and allow to cool completely on a metal cooling rack before slicing into 10 slices.

Made in the USA
Columbia, SC
22 August 2021